V I G I L

THE POETRY OF PRESENCE

Pamela Heinrich MacPherson

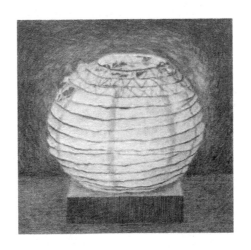

V I G I L

THE POETRY OF PRESENCE

Pamela Heinrich MacPherson

Vigil: The Poetry of Presence
Poems by Pamela Heinrich MacPherson
Copyright 2016 by Pamela Heinrich MacPherson
Cover illustration and design by Carol E.S. MacDonald. www.CarolMacDonald.com
Photo of author by Andrew L. MacPherson
Chapter illustrations by Pamela Heinrich MacPherson
Permission has been granted for use of quotes on chapter pages.

ISBN: 9780692777619

CONTACT:
Pamela Heinrich MacPherson
South Burlington, VT 05403
vigilthepoetryofpresence@gmail.com

Acknowledgements

I am profoundly grateful to Sue Brooks
for her insightful wisdom, guidance and loving support.

I extend heartfelt appreciation to Zail Berry,
Judy Lief, Camilla Rockwell and Don Schumacher for reading this
manuscript and offering endorsements.

My deepest gratitude is extended to my dearest ones
for their unconditional love and belief in me.

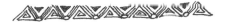

This book is dedicated to all of my teachers
in the lessons of living and of dying.

If I can stop one heart from breaking
I shall not live in vain;
If I can ease one life the aching,
Or cool one pain,
Or help one fainting robin
Unto his nest again,
I shall not live in vain.

Emily Dickinson

x

CONTENTS

PREFACE

"We have a woman who is alone and dying. Any time that
you can give will be appreciated. Call me and I'll give you
details." The richness and fullness of my own life dims...
someone is dying and is alone. One of the most profound
experiences of life is occurring and I have the opportunity to
be present. Within a few hours, in the dark of late evening,
I enter the hospital room of a stranger, ready to leave the
outside world behind; ready to open my heart.

*Vigil: Latin: Vigilo "to be awake", be vigilant; a period of
watchful attention; wakefulness that holds calm; bearing quiet
solemn witness.*

It is a privilege to bear witness to the sacred process of dying.
Each individual with whom I sit vigil is unique; every situation
different. Leaving my own life and doings at the door, I enter
the room silently naming my intention: to be fully present
to whatever awaits me. I gently introduce myself, whether
the individual appears aware or not, and offer my presence.
During the next few hours, as I sit quietly at the bedside, my
instinct may tell me to gently touch, hum softly, match my
breathing to theirs or simply sit close, perhaps occasionally
softly speaking words of encouragement and affirmation.

Writing poetry is my manner of processing. In many aspects of my life, poetry and writing are how I sift and grow through what I am experiencing; it seems to be the way my brain is wired. Being able to express myself with an economy of words, whether from a place of doubt or distress, delight, or a desire to preserve my experience, I am transported to a place of greater understanding and deeper appreciation. I neither seek critique nor need approval. When I write from an open heart, my soul becomes visible.

The poems in this book flow from the sacred moments of sitting vigil. They have lived, in my handwriting, in a private journal dedicated to my vigil-sitting experiences. This was my safe place for processing; my haven for unfiltered, unedited writing. These works were never written with the intention of being published. However, now, in my eighth decade, I have begun to think about what of mine I want to preserve for our children. In reviewing my journals, this poetry felt worthy. And then, when I read a few to close friends, their passionate response sealed my commitment to share them with a wider audience.

I didn't anticipate the feelings that would come when I lifted the poems from their private, personal place in my journal and exposed them in typed format on stark white paper. Without my handwriting, they felt altered, diminished, somehow less intimate. This experience held an unexpected lesson for me. There was a sense of letting go that urged me to trust and accept whatever happened next... perhaps, I mused, not unlike the dying process itself.

In time, it came to me that my meditation candle, a small votive within a paper globe, was the perfect image for the cover of this book. Envisioning the candle causes me to take a slow deep breath and begin to lean toward quiet and centering. When I was shown the initial sketch of the image, I asked my dear friend Carol, the artist who rendered it, if the tattered and worn area of the globe would be best "neatened up" a bit. She responded with great insight, "Pam, both life and death have their tatters. It needs to stay as it is." Ahhh... she was so right.

No matter how busy I am, when I take the time to say "yes" to a vigil request, I am rewarded with exposure to some of the most sacred spaces in life – bearing witness to the dying process... a body and spirit pulling into center, a world becoming smaller as a spirit expands and prepares for its release from its corporal housing.

And, when I am in what feels like a long dry spell from vigil requests, I sometimes (selfishly perhaps) yearn for the call to sit with someone who is dying. When my own life is too full and I am feeling worn, I realize that what has been missing is the quiet of connecting with my own soul. While what I give when I sit vigil is genuine and intuitive in the moment, what I receive transforms me, brings me to my silent center of peace. The opportunity to enter a room and consciously empty myself of all that is outside the room – to be fully present to the solemn and profound final moments in the lifetime of another – is a sacred gift.

In the Hospice tradition, as with all healthcare settings, confidentiality is always respected. Vigil sitting experiences are no exception. In these works, I have changed names and altered recognizable characteristics and situations to keep the identity of all I serve in confidence. An exception has been made in Chapter 9 where the permission of the families has been obtained.

CHAPTER 1

Presence

"Those who have the strength and the love to sit with a dying patient in the silence that goes beyond words will know that this moment is neither frightening, nor painful, but a peaceful cessation of the functioning of the body."

ELISABETH KÜBLER-ROSS

Soul Gifts

The gift of time,
Of silence,
The practice of presence,
Listening…
Giving dignity, respect and compassion
To each dying person,
As I sit alone sharing sacred passing moments.

Gentle touch,
Soft reassurance,
My small gifts to give
As I bear witness…
As I am being with…

Gifts from the soul:
Time and presence.

Hands

Hands so soft.
Hands that held a fork,
That caressed a lover…
Hands that toiled in work
And waved a warm greeting…

Hands so soft…
That wiped a falling tear
And were held by a loving mother–
And now they are still.

Hands that cast a vote
And gripped a steering wheel.
Hands that greeted a stranger
And lifted a wee one.
Hands that swam in water
And shivered in winter
Hands that now lay still.

Yes, those imprints of greeting,
Of loving, of toiling,
Of sustaining, of reaching
Leave their mark on the lives of others.

Is that a form of afterlife?

With certainty!

Escape

Silent deep sleep,
The blessing of drugs
To calm a disturbed, restless soul.

Soft music…
And your companion pussycat
Loving my caresses
And pawing my pen as I write.

Sleep troubled dear one.
Let sleep's escape bring you peace
In this, the journey of your lifetime.

Leave peacefully
Destined for places of greater happiness.

Softest Hands; Softest Ears

Suddenly…
Life on the brink –
Scott and Jo's sweet woofer, Lexi,
Is found to be filled with cancer.

And you, dear one,
Your hospital stay tragically detoured
By a sudden internal event
That places you in a coma.

These two worlds collide in mine.
It is your silky soft hand
That I hold, that I gently caress,
That brings my thoughts to Lexi,
A beloved beagle
About whom, I have always said,
I log the softest ears on the planet!

My hands have glided lovingly
On the smooth, warm, satiny surface of both.
Will your two worlds intersect?
Will Lexi,
Who left this world just six days ago,
Await your arrival,
You bringing your soft gentle hand
To rub those brown silky triangular ears?

What an unconditionally loving
And tail-wagging welcome that would be!

Dona Nobis Pacem

Cachectic, sunken…
His body ready to dismiss
His spirit, loved by all.

Late at night
I arrive in the low-lit hospital room
Of a single, fifth-decade gent
Cared for by loving parents
For far too many years to mention.
A twisted, contractured body
Does not define this man.
Even in his dying days
His glowing spirit and courage
Are clear evidence
Of the sound foundation
Of his earthly existence.

Boney prominences,
Sunken cavities,
Organs protein-scarred.
Yet he is upbeat… brave…
Has lived a good life,
One he's sad to leave.

His Catholic faith
Is not only intact
But is the source of his strength.
It's late evening,
He closes and then opens his eyes.

Sitting next to him,
I lean in and, in the darkness,
Begin to softly hum
Every Catholic hymn and chant
I can think of
From my far and distant past.

His eyes close.
He settles.

May he be aware
That a place of perfect peace awaits him.

ICU

Lines, tubes, numbers…
Flashing, rolling, beeping…
Digits rising,
Numbers falling.
Half-mast eyes partially open,
Lids slowly lower
A sea of equipment his view.

"Vanco on"…
A digitalized screen announces
The presence of an antibiotic.
Dialysis continues,
Pumping out and returning warm blood
Flowing through narrow tubing channels
Removing excess fluids
And bloodstream wastes.

Mechanical navigational charts
Cleansing,
Stabilizing,
Maintaining
Your body, outside your body.

I sit near, yet feeling far.

How I want to fluff your pillow
And position your weakened body
Until you nod a nod of comfort
And drift off to peaceful sleep.

I can only hold your hand
And send you mental energy
For comfort – and healing –
And relief.

Soul Friend

In a peaceful, still, lowly-lit room
Lies a gentle man,
A stranger to me,
Who, by choice,
Had the ventilator
That assisted his trach'ed breathing,
Removed …
An act of both courage and sensibility.

He now rests tranquilly,
Away from intensive care
In a private room
Having accepted
And now allowing
The natural, gradual, slow release
Of worn out and challenged
Basic life-holding body systems.

Presence is what I offer.
Unconditional acceptance,
Deep respect,
Compassionate caring.

Our unspoken connection
Rises from the heart.
Within moments,
As I settle in next to him,
He becomes a soul-friend.

I'll Be Right Here

Soft spoken,
Though a bit raspy,
His exhausted body
Sits upright and blanket-wrapped
In a chair next to his bed.
His eyes are closed
To the room and to the reality.
His head slowly droops,
Spoken word stopped mid-sentence;
Chin lowers,
A short snooze of a minute or two,
Then, as head rises quickly,
His breathing escalates.
He focuses on his breath.

I sit next to him, my hand on his arm
And find my softest, most lulling voice...

"You're tired," I say. "Let it happen."
"I know, but I can't..."
"Is this new?" I ask.
"No."
"Are you afraid to fall asleep?"
"I think so."
Do you know what you're afraid of?"
"No ..."

"Well, I'll be right here.
Focus on your breathing.
Picture a beautiful calm ocean.
Each breath is like a wave,
Gently ride on each wave."

I promise…
"I'll be right here."

Angst

Moaning…
What is your angst?
How can we tell
Existential from physical?

Pain in any form
Is unacceptable.

We'll try.
You join us in trying.
Perhaps…

Peace awaits.

I Am Just Going to Hold Your Hand

"I am just going to hold your hand."
How many times have I said that,
Offering to sit silently
At the bedside,
To just be there…
"You may sleep."

"I'm just going to hold your hand,"
Said high school freshman, Benny,
As we sat awkwardly silent
On the living room couch,
Him a secret intruder
After two-year old Kolleen,
Whom I was babysitting,
Had gone to sleep for the night.
This, the timid, tongue tied silence
Of my first dating experience.

Now, those words
Glide over my lips so easily…
Always spoken from my heart,
They are permission,
A promise of presence,
Focused attendance
In bearing witness.

And while silence is golden,
I am now neither tongue-tied
Nor timid about opening my heart
To these precious, sacred moments
Shared with another.

Playing Through

(I arrived to sit vigil with very little information about this gentleman. My cues must come from objects in the room.)

A grandfather,
A shelved photo of
Four cherubic faces reveals.
But what else?

Little evidence in this room
Of machinery noises
As you sleep your way to death.
But wait!
I did see golf clubs
Imprinted on your door's nameplate.

Hands still, positioned by others.
Hands that once held a tight grip.

What else?
Did you yell, "Fore!"?
Are you calling that out now
So others will get out of the way?
Perhaps they will stand and bear witness
To this, your greatest shot
On the 18th hole of life.

CHAPTER 2
Being of Use

*"It is one of the most beautiful compensations
of life – no man can sincerely try to help
another without helping himself."*

RALPH WALDO EMERSON

Is It Time?

"Is it time?"
His eyes close and he wonders…
Weakened voice;
Deep, painful cough.
He returns
From a brief semi-awake moment
To the shallow sleep
That permeates his current status.

Five days ago,
Such a short time
And yet a rich deep time
In our new relationship.
A request came to me
From the Hospice Volunteer Office…
A volunteer to preserve his "story."
"Time is short."
"He's a great storyteller!"
And indeed, 'twas true.

Only four daily visits
And each day
On my late afternoon arrival, I am warned,
"He's had a bad day."
"He's slept most of the day."

His family leaves the room, as we had agreed,
I arrange my chair next to his bed,
Prepare my voice recorder and,
Gently touching his shoulder, I say his name.

His eyes open
And honestly have a twinkle.
He softly greets me, knowing my mission.
I ask if he'd like to do more reminiscing with me.
With his positive nod,
I clip the tiny microphone on him and say:
"Tell me about your Mother,"
And we're off….

So it was for four visits.
My concern about tiring him
Was met with denial.

"I remember her kitchen,"
The story begins…
And stretches to an older brother,
"My protector when I was bullied at school…"
Each day brings forth remembered times
Full of richness and detail.
Parents, grandparents and siblings
Are all described and woven into
Tales of childhood adventures
And parochial school days.

"My wife....
She's the best thing that ever happened to me,"
He tenderly shares.
Pride in their children's accomplishments
Extend down through young adult grandchildren.
Photos come out,
More stories flow
And his saddest admission is shared:
"I never told my children I loved them enough."
"I'm learning to do it now...."
His voice trails off emotionally.
"It's so hard to leave them...."

The fifth day,
With the same arrival status shared,
I settle in, touch his shoulder,
And say his name.
But it was different.
"Shall we try?" I ask.
He opens his eyes, nods,
And then dozes off again.

There was to be no more.
While I had captured over five hours,
His storytelling was done.
I sat with him, held his hand
And one time when he awoke
He asked me if it was time.
I said the time was getting closer.

I assured him there was time…
Time for him to receive more love from his family;
Time for him to lean into peaceful sleep;
"Someone will always be with you," I promised.

I thanked him for his gift of friendship
And promised him the stories he shared with me
Will be preserved for his family;
"This is another way you will be present with them,"
I promised,
As in the bountiful tomorrows
They lovingly hold his gentle spirit
With them….
Forevermore.

Midnight Moment

Eyes open
Staring
Blinking
Half-mast after Morphine…
But seeing?

Faintest of bare nod
When asked yes or no,
Mouth agape
Body still
But eyes staring.

I speak your name.
I touch you
And turn on soft music I brought.
I rub your arm; hold your hand.
No response,
But I trust you know.

Then at midnight,
I tell you I must leave
And have to take my music.
Your eyes turned right to me!
Oh no… You liked it.
I hate to take it
So I make arrangements
For a CD player and music
To be brought to your bedside.

You never know…

Socks Rock!

"I'm freezing…", she mutters.
And her hands are, indeed.

Every thirty to forty-five seconds
Arms reach out. Flail.
"I'm freezing…", she repeats.

We hold hands,
Warming under the covers,
Touching, rubbing,
All to no relief,
Though feeling warmer to me.

Pattern continues.
Finally at ten o'clock I get the idea…
Hospital socks!

"I know what we can do.
One minute, dear…"
I am thinking:
I'll get some pretty blue ones.
Soon her hands are encased.
Voila! Soft mitties!
She slowly settles into sleep.

I feel fatigue creeping in
The hour is late.
Our third-born arrives on a late flight tonight.
I'll go to meet him when I leave.

Good night, dear and fragile one.
Stay warm in peaceful sleep.
May angels soon come
And warmly bring you home.

Midnight Move

Calm… Quiet… Settled.
It's almost as if she is reflecting
In the calm, orderly, quiet environment
Nurse Kathleen has created.

She is responsive, though medicated.
Purple hands evidence her painful journey
Through medicated care.

We connect…
She holds my hands,
Actually my scarf, too.
Tight.
"What can I do?" she asks twice.
Restless, she is pleading.
Kathleen reassures and then medicates her.
I hold her hand and give her ginger ale.
Other caring staff, when restlessness persists,
Turn and reposition her.
Thankfully, she slowly fades
To medication-induced sleep.

The charge nurse beckons me to the hallway.
He is very upset.
"They want to move her."
"Patients in the ER need beds;
I fought it – it's wrong", he continued
"To move her at this point."
"Where?", I ask.
"Shep 4, Oncology. They know comfort care."
"I fought administration," he tells me.
"We do this work because we care…
And we do it well."
His frustrated, teary, voice trails off….

"I will stay to help smooth the transfer," I offer,
Even though past my assigned time.
"It must be done quietly, gently.
And it must be a quiet room, if not private.
She's just settled down," I advocate.
"Thank you. Thank you." he responds.

Oh my… how unfortunate.
But we must think of those waiting in the ER.
My friend Carol was one of those not too long ago.
"With this woman's move," I offer,
"They gain two beds."
"Thank you for reminding me of that," he replies.

CHAPTER 3
Bearing Witness

*"When we bear witness, when we become
the situation … the right action arises by itself.
We don't have to worry about what to do. We don't
have to figure out solutions ahead of time …
Once we listen with our entire body
and mind, loving action arises."*

BERNIE GLASSMAN

Hallowed Hallway

A name
Sounding vaguely familiar
And a room number
("But he's being transferred," I am told)
What new experience awaits me
In the sacred territory of dying?

As I enter the hospital,
Moving through long winding hallways,
Faces pass me,
Concerned loved ones easily identified.
Other countenances, with focused expressions,
Hurry to their next destination.

Oh hallowed hallways
And rabbit warren chambers,
You bear witness
To days and nights of joy and sorrow –
Fears of diagnosis,
Apprehensions for treatment,
Families sitting vigil with dying loved ones –
All intervals of uncertainty,
While above, on the next floor,
A joyful new life begins…

This medical center:
One vast vessel holding the fullness of life,
Balancing beginnings and endings
And all the challenges of health-filled existence
In the moments, days, months and years
That lie in between.

Birth Love

Flashing through the window,
Passing car light beams
Glisten on the rain-slick street,
A reminder of life as usual
While one small frail woman
Sleeps the gentle sleep
Of a Morphine drip.

A motionless body
Winding down,
Her corporal mechanisms
Overworked, worn out,
Challenged by alcohol
To the point of failure.
Fifty-five mortal years
Closing in,
Preparing to release a spirit
For whom, I sense,
Life was not fair.

May she have felt loved.
May some of her wishes have come true.
May she have laughed heartily
And been embraced
When overcome with sadness and tears.

In this moment
I will hold her parents' love for her
On the day she was born,
Returning it to her
Through my compassionate presence,
As I witness her final hours and moments
In this universe that is all we know.

Work Boots Tell a Story

Angular, narrow, mustached face
Rhythmical breathing of medicated body
That six days ago
Was up and fighting to go home.
Heavy black work boots stand motionless in the corner.
One holds a brace to minimize a limp that,
Along with years of unrelenting hip pain,
Echoes the ramifications of a teenage car accident.

All aspects of life were interfered with,
Inhibited by and diminished by
The dark shadows of challenged health.

With me, a gentle loving brother sits across the bed
And shares soft-spoken stories
Of his brother's love of fishing…
A man whose physical limitations
Made him sit in a chair streamside –
Limited his ability to have regular meaningful work-
Cast a dark shadow on his potential.

This man drew the short straw in life;
Yet, in the eyes of his accomplished brother,
He is loved, appreciated and valued for what's inside…
Remnants of a childhood, evidence of family values…
Their Mom and Dad would be proud.

Presence

Presence with touch…
With voice…
Bearing witness.
One soul
Moving toward forever.

I have only a name
As I gently rub her shoulder
To message my presence.
Attentively I listen
To the short even breaths
Through a gaping mouth,
Counting down the hours
Until only her shell remains,
The husk that for sixty-eight years
Held her now-releasing spirit.

Be at peace.
Let go… release.
Soar, dear soul.

Whose Son Is This?

Whose son is this?
Whose innocent babe grown homeless?
What life path divided
At perhaps a critical time,
Mental illness guiding his itinerary
Through troubled decades…
A schizophrenic burden his to carry.

As I hold his hand
Reading my book of Silence
His breathing stops…
Ever so quietly.
This gentle soundless exit is,
Truly, the ultimate silence.

Bearing witness,
I lean in and softly say:
Go – Go to your mother.
She awaits you,
Her child who had such a difficult life.
Fly, spirit…
You are now free.

I wonder...
Is his spirit soul gone?
I see his shell,
Feel the slowly creeping in coldness.
Silence of spirit, now of body.
Silence.
Freedom....

Waiting

I must wait for the obituary
To learn the values, the passions,
The vocations and the family
Of this one who appears so loved
And now, is a silent shell
In the darkness of this silent night
Lying in wait for death.

I am here to simply bear witness
To human withering,
Respect his uniqueness
And be present to the process
So he is not alone
In this, his final chapter.

Still Point

Me,
A stranger at your bedside,
Your hand held in mine as,
In this stilled, dimly lit space
That is your hospital room,
I breathe with you,
Matching my breath
To your shallow, fading air exchange.

How could I know
What I was about to receive?
Your presence, your dying,
Brings me to my still point,
The place of centering and calm
So difficult to access
In the hum and buzz of everyday living,
A place where nothing exists
Beyond our sacred, shared presence.

To not die alone,
To bear witness to this sacred transition,
To stand in for all who ever loved you –
A privilege beyond description.

Spirit
Be free…
Fly in the space of complete peace
And be held in the all-accompanying embrace
Of all loving ancestors.

CHAPTER 4
Process

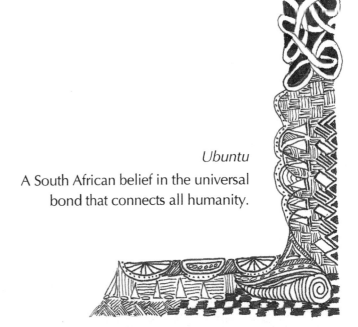

Ubuntu
A South African belief in the universal
bond that connects all humanity.

In An Instant Life Changes

Medical ICU
A robust looking, sturdy man,
Ready to ambulate this morning
When…. POOF!
An internal crisis
Robbed him of all possibility.

Husky and healthy looking
Man of six decades –
Truck driver, farmer…
Whatever his labor…
I imagine him to have worked hard,
Attended the School of Hard Knocks
And to have been no stranger to struggles.
Two small photos of grandchildren
Propped in his lifeless hand,
Tell of family not immediately present.

May he have felt the joy of their love,
The loyalty of good friends
And satisfaction with his labors.

Your earthly work is done, my friend.
May you be at peace.
May this world be a better place
Because you were a part of it.

Giving Time

What magnetic pull
Does this earthly existence have?
What power? What reason?

This spirit seems ready to go
Yet a strong fifty year old body
Allows time for those for whom this loss
Will be felt for all time to come.

May the spirit leaving
And the hands and hearts that must remain
Be in concert,
Embracing each other,
Bidding sweet farewell
At the magical, sacred, mystical
Moment of passage

To forevermore…

Life Interrupted

Hold on tight and let go…
The Ying and Yang of dying.

You lie in wait
With no response now…
Skin paper-thin,
Appearing violated by treatments.
Your time is here.
Yet in this our first meeting,
You seem so not ready.

Near your bed I see…
Current magazines,
Well-worn address book,
Recent Miles Kimball catalog,
Mail looking like you just read it.
Your nails are painted
And snacks lie waiting nearby.

It is now,
Following a sudden unexplained internal event,
That you will leave all behind.
The intensive care of this unit
Is unable to make the difference.
Your family is grieving deeply.

Your other family of ancestors awaits…
May their embrace fill your cup
With perfect love and peace.

Being Present Doesn't Feel Like Enough

Portly, burly
Man of limited days…
How can I help you?

I speak my name
Hold your hand in both of mine
But you are restless –
Rapid mouth breathing;
Head and arms rest
Then turn and flail.
Your racing pulse
Throbs in your vessels,
Blood flow bouncing
On the precarious
Trampoline of life.

We await your next dose of Morphine.
Ativan Is slipped In intravenously.
"There are technical problems,"
Your nurse announces,
About obtaining your prescribed Morphine.

Your pulse races at 140;
A mini belly convulsion
Pulls each breath in.
Heaving… releasing….

Are you afraid?
What are you feeling?
Your color grays.
Someone will be with you.
Be restful.
Lean into the hidden cave of sleep.
Perhaps there,
You can find your elusive place of peace.

Drugs

Damn that we need them.
Bless that we have them.

Mama Waits

Responsive.
Anxious.
Adult child and spouse left today.

Expiratory moans…
Fear, anxiety, isolation observed.
Meds given for relief.
Hand resting on favorite soft stuffed dog.

"Anna" – I softly speak her name.
Aware when awake,
Though in and out of sleep
Through medicated blessings.
"Sleep like your doggie, dear.

He'll always stay at your side.
May you sleep
As peacefully as he does."

"Mama…"
Breath in, pause…
Breath out.

"Mama…."
Breath in, pause…
Breath out,
"Mama…"

"I feel her holding you, Anna…
Know how much she loves you."
"*Yes.*"

"Is she waiting for you?"
"*Yes…*"

"Where?"
"*Somewhere…*"

"Go to the place where she waits, Anna.
I must leave now;
I'll hold you in my thoughts.
You can go to Mama.
Mama loves you.
Mama waits for you."

Is It Ready?

A gentle loving daughter
Is ever-present,
Your loving companion
On your journey of dying.

You rub your leg, reaching,
Your catheter just out of reach.
Arm extends skyward,
Your hand returning to
Patterned rubbing of your leg.
"Okay," you say, repeatedly
As you pick at your nightgown.
"Okay? Is it ready?"

Then you enter ten snoring minutes,
Your brief escape from uncertainty,
Blessed refuge from restless picking.
You can leave, dear.
Everyone will be okay.
Your long life is ending.
Find peace.
Be at rest.

Indeed, yes. "It is ready."

Nothing Dignified

There is nothing dignified
About teeth being out,
The urgency of a bowel movement,
Flatulence released,
Ecchymotic hands that are
The extension of tissue paper arms.

A woman cries out…

"Are you in pain?"
"*Yes*"
"Where?"
A muffled, "*All over.*"
At least that's what it sounded like.

I call for the nurse.

No –
Nothing dignified in this dying.

May a warm hand on hers be felt.
May her passage come soon.
I want more for her.
She deserves better.

Midnight Vigil

Unshaven, balding…
Twitching and occasional reaching out
A light restlessness –

"Was he turned?" I ask.
Nurse: "I took his pillow out."
He's been here for about a year.
Oh my…
Dialysis discontinued six days ago.
Each inhale ends in a gentle gurgle.

The March wind howls
Through trees, around buildings…
A warm midnight wind
That will caress my body when I leave,
My grateful, able, life-engaged body.

But first –
Sleep, my friend.
Find a peaceful place.
Rest bones weary from illness.
Travel chemically to a place of peace.
Your tough journey is almost complete.

You are at the finish line.
This day is moments away from being done.

Nursing Home Years

Part I

My alarm sounds at 5am.
As advised, I call in to check.
"Yes, do please come,
She is still with us."

Early morning light begins to dawn;
Yellow-grey smoky sky holds random clouds and,
As darkness lifts,
I am aware that a soul is also preparing to rise
To its self-chosen new life.

I exit the elevator.
A warm woman with a Cape Verdian accent greets me:
"Good morning; thank you for coming."
She escorts me to the room.

"She's not breathing like she was," she quickly observes
And with a questioning eye
And a hand-seeking pulse,
We both realize that this long-term elder
Has just passed.
She promptly leaves seeking a nurse.

As there is another elder, a roommate,
Behind the curtain in the other bed,
I dim the light, raise the bed
And settle at its side to await a nurse's pronouncement.
My hand caresses her lifeless arm
As I softly hum "Amazing Grace"
Wishing her peace on her soul journey.

Her body is still warm,
Color only beginning to be drawn
From her soft, age-wrinkled face.
A favorite doll lays cuddled at her side.

Be well
And be whole in a new way.
Your long nursing home years
Are now behind you.

Nursing Home Roommates

Nursing Home Years, Part II

How is it,
During sleep assigned hours
To listen to
The rhythmic gurgle
And gradual slowing
Of your roommate's breathing?

Then there is silence.

No one is present,
Yet you heard the moment,
The passage
From sound to silence,
A transition so smooth,
Without struggle,
Appearing to be without witness.

Were you awake?
Were you aware?
Is this one more roommate leaving?

Are you comforted
By how naturally and gently
This transition occurred,
Knowing someday…

I wish to hold your hand for a minute
And let you know
That I understand, I care,
And that I am grateful
That you were present.

Winding Down

The work of breathing,
The last task of living…
Rhythmic – automatic
While sleep prevails,
Is central,
Whether natural
Or chemically-induced.
The corporal machinery winds down
Ever so slowly,
First shutting down more distant
And less critical mechanisms,
Until only the essential workings
Of the heart and lungs remain.

Time.
It takes time.

An open-hearted, focused presence
Is what we can bring,
A compassionate and loving gift
In these last days, hours and moments.
It is all.
It is sacred.
It is enough….

CHAPTER 5
Quality of Care

"Learn to get in touch with the silence within yourself and know that everything in this life has a purpose; there are no mistakes, no coincidences, all events are blessings given to us to learn from."

ELISABETH KÜBLER-ROSS

Best Care Possible

The residents on duty
Have spoken with the family.
Their advice and guidance
Has been met with religion-based resistance.

Decisions around the use of medications
And intravenous fluids,
When using the words
Hastening and *prolonging,*
Often are based in fear and emotion.
Religion and fear can so get in the way
Of compassionate decisions.

It is a very wise and skilled professional
That can facilitate a discussion,
Assisting emotional family members
In understanding the tenets
Of compassionate end-of-life care.

To honor an organic, natural process,
While expressing love, giving thanks
And being fully present
In the final hours of life's journey
Is, indeed, the best care possible.

Care: Acceptance on My Part

Tiny and frail and barely a shadow of who she was,
This nonagenarian's petite features
Are immersed deeply in somnolence.

I touch her shoulder and speak her name...
No response.

Discolored hands tell of medical misfortune.
Sleep is deep as rhythmic air passes through open
orifice.
I sit, touching purple hands,
Thinking of what she has been through.

Oh no... I notice that her sheet is wet.
Her intravenous is leaking.
It's then that my eyes rest on a very swollen arm.

Finding her nurse in the hallway,
I tell of my concern
"It can't be," he quickly responds.
"Did you touch it?" he defensively questions.
I simply state my request again –
"Will you please check her I/V?"
And turn to return to the room.
Realizing his accusation,
He shifts and thanks me for noticing.

He arrives in the room,
Examines her arm and intravenous site.
"Another must be placed," he announces.
"Her family wants it," he defends…
This sentence is hard for me to hear;
My heart questions.
Her family? What about her wishes?
I remind myself that my role is presence…
My reluctant mind strains for acceptance.

Later, a very skilled I/V nurse met with success
Puncturing the bruised, tissue-thin skin
In this apneic ninety-three year old.

I am feeling helpless.
I remind myself that touch and expressed caring
Have immeasurable potential.
I focus on being present.
My touch and voice tell that I care.
Indeed, I do…

Mediocre

Mediocre…
A level of nursing care
Not without polite exchanges
Or meeting basic needs.

However,
Absent was a lingering touch that knows,
Bending to the patient's equal level,
The turning of a too-warm pillow,
Moistening lips with more than oil
But also with caring words
That moisten the dying soul.

Presence is more than the opposite of absence;
One can be recognizably absent
When fully physically present.

My lesson last night
Was in the recognition of mediocrity.
On paper, everything would appear fine.
In person,
Compassion and soul were absent.

My helplessness,
In the face of knowing what was missing
And wishing to provide it,
Leaves me grieving her last hours and moments.
They were so full of absence.

I do not wish to judge.

From observing and processing,
I am committed to sharpening my insight
And deepening my understanding.
There are lessons I am to learn
And carry forward.

Turning Up the Dial on Compassionate Care

There are so many ways for life to feel not fair.
No one is necessarily to blame;
Nothing was actually done wrong.

Let's face it:
Care does exist
That only rises to mediocre on the dial.
Some nurses are just better than others.

And the next night,
Sitting with the same patient,
My care scorecard becomes balanced
As I witness a new nurse
Giving beautiful, compassionate, attentive care
Moving the dial all the way up to "what you deserve."

Relief

Low level agitation.
Twitching. Reaching.
Awake.
Christmas Eve dawns.
You, three days away
From completing your 89th year…
Me, not knowing you –
Your baseline,
Not liking how restless you are.

Twitches, both voluntary and involuntary.
"Do you have pain," I ask?
"No."
"How can I make you more comfortable?"
No answer…
The night nurse enters
With precaution gown half askew.
Ativan is placed under your tongue.
Your eyes are open
"He sleeps with his eyes open," she shares.
She leaves.

"What are you thinking about?" I inquire.
Your one word answer: "Life."
Restlessness persists.

An hour later your day nurse arrives.
She greets you affectionately.
She is so knowing, and caring.
She tells me you came in two days ago
And were sleeping all the time.
"I see the changes today," she offers.
Leaving briefly,
She returns with a swifter acting medication.
Sleep comes quickly.

Finally,
Your twitching and restlessness is relieved.
She checks frequently;
She knows and acts.
She exudes compassionate care.

You are in good hands now.

Obstacles

I arrive at 9pm.
A white-haired, chemically-unresponsive woman
Lies quietly, breathing her last breaths.
In her hospital room, florescent lights glare
And noisy radio is tuned to 106.7,
The Wizard of Rock station.
Oh my….

"I was told that's what she wants,"
The volunteer shares with me

> *Rock music blocks silence;*
> *Bright lights are a salve for fear.*

The other volunteer leaves,
I settle in
In a room of random-turned broken shade slats,
Surfaces strewn with medical supplies.
False teeth and toiletries
Lay among tubes, bandages and stray ephemera.
I touch her arm – share that I'll be at her bedside.
I witness breaths – labored,
Seeking more air.

> *Chatty radio hosts*
> *Are using words like bitch and other offensives*
> *In their one-upping each other diatribe…*

A nurse comes in, observes,
Decides not to re-medicate yet.
I sit, touch and hope.
I want to breathe for her.

> *"Sex toys, women get more benefit,*
> *Makes it hard for men to please". They go on…*

The rock music, I now realize,
Actually is becoming my respite
From their edgy, objectionable topics.

She stirs, is restless. I give reassurance
And can see it's not enough.
I ring for the nurse as she moves, turns,
And can't find a place of relief.

> *Guitars squeal; drums pound.*

Please come, I mentally beg,
This woman is reaching, needing.
I go to the door and signal a nurse.
Nursing verbal reassurance, however,
Brings no relief when you're struggling to breathe.
Morphine is administered by I/V, then Ativan.
Soon the patient begins to settle,
Though there is still great effort in breathing.

Two hours have passed. It is 11pm
And breathing, while asleep, is still labored.
"I'll get Respiratory Therapy to do a nebulizer,"
The absent-for-long-stretches nurse says,
Seeming, in my eyes,
Inexperienced in powerful comfort measures.
She hasn't turned and positioned her –
Changed her wet-from-sweat pillow
Or done any gentle, comfort-for-the-dying measures.
Nice enough gal;
Perhaps overextended with patient assignments.
No eye (or time) for detail nor ability to be soul-present.

It's 11:40pm now and this dear woman has died…
Actually about twenty minutes ago.
I am now sitting in the empty hospital lobby
In a private, quiet spot where I can process.

Suffering is what I witnessed
Breathing that gasped for more air for hours…
Medication not sufficient to alleviate;
A nurse not skilled enough or intuitive enough
To give the best care possible.

No words of comfort or blessing
As this dear woman passed –
Only rigid silence – Feeling for a pulse –
A hand that could have comforted or caressed,
Chose to freeze in a pulse-checking position.

I knew better. I unobtrusively reached in.
My two hands held her hand
As I told her we were with her,
Offered a blessing that she find peace.
I felt very inhibited, limited.
I didn't feel I could reach beyond,
Upstaging the nurse.

I am so sorry, so very sorry.
I held your soul in my heart
And could only, silently,
Wish you journey blessings.
I am tearful.
I am deeply saddened
By my blocked ineffectiveness,
The sterility of your closure,
And my inability to be more present to you.

I left as quietly as I arrived,
Carrying your suffering as my grief.

CHAPTER 6
Growth

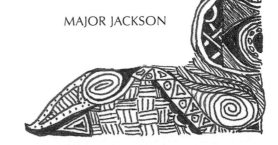

*"It's a belief in writing poetry as a spiritual,
life-giving practice, where breathing and
contemplating inside language attunes
us to a greater self and awareness."*

MAJOR JACKSON

My Morrie

Ever so still –
Clock ticking,
City lights reflecting in living room,
The hum of passing traffic,
Morning light reflected off Huntington bricks.
I am in the darkened small-world room
Of a sage old man.
"I'm from New York,"
Spills from white-mustached lips.
"I've been all over;
 I've done it all..."
His New York accented voice
Trails off into memories.

The TV is on with the sound muted,
"The best way to hear the news," he offers
With a twinkle in his sleepy eyes.
He leans in and out of brief naps.

This man could be my teacher,
My Tuesdays with Morrie;
A weekly dose of sage wisdom.
But that gift will be given
To the volunteer who, today, I am replacing
And I'll hope for an occasional dose.

He asks about my parents, their work…
I was proud to speak of my Dad.
"He was a good man," I share,
Without a tear or sadness.
"I miss him," I say tenderly,
Not mentioning his death being merely months before.
Healing has occurred; it is taking time…
The path known to others, now new to me.

I was immediately aware
Of how far my grieving process has come.
While I had accepted Dad's death,
There was a large hole in my world.

I sense that if I shared this with my Morrie
His advice would be grounding, affirming, wise.
But I won't. This isn't about me.
However, I am touched by his thoughtfulness,
His inquiry into my world;
A generous, kind spirit
Taking a part of me into his shrinking sphere.

Mechanical

It's the night before New Year's Eve.
One more assignment.
My usual 9pm to midnight.
And I sit.

I am present physically
However, that seems to be all.

A former machinist, I am told.
Breathing
Pulsating
Flaccid
Medicated
Life now measured in hours.

I assist the nurse in turning him
Laying fresh sheets
And positioning him to what looks comfortable
Then I sit.

Mechanical breathing,
Thready pulse,
His only connections to life.
And I sit.

I touch and speak.
I give permission to let go.
I remind that there are many who love him.
But I don't feel soul-connection.

Am I getting shop worn?

So Long

So long it has been
To witness dying…
Me a caring stranger;
You on life's most meaningful voyage.

Teach me.
Help me to live in the present,
Value each moment,
Remember our mortal limits
As, some day
In living into my future,
I will exist as you do now,
One foot on terra (not so) firma,
The other dangling over the precipice
That holds time eternal.

Move forward on your journey.
Loosen your grasp on here and now.
You can do it, my friend.
Let your spirit rise
And your physical body fall.

So long….

Magnificent View; End of Hallway

Cold December darkness
Surrounds my 6am arrival.
Together, we'll watch night
Draw open the curtains of dawn.

In this, the newest building
Of our medical center complex,
A nurse ushers me to your room,
The last one at the end of the hall.

I can't help remembering Kubler-Ross,
In her culture-changing book,
Telling of dying patients in the 1950's
Being placed in a room
That was furthest from the nurses station.
Those death-denying days
Found the dying dismissed
In favor of the living.

I mention this as a recollection,
The young nurse quickly responds saying,
"Oh, we turn him every three hours
And we give him mouth care."
She goes on…
I realized she's too young to know
A time, decades ago, in which I nursed.

You are gifted a magnificent view
Overlooking our beautiful Queen City.
The college chapel spire
Points like a glistening beacon
To the waiting heavens above.
In the distance, Water Tower Hill
Is barely discernable
In the grey, turning-blue morning mist.

Morning rounds begin
And the hospital comes alive.
Your doctor visits,
Observes you breathing easily,
Seeming comfortable and pain free.
He nods his approval
And his white coat turns the corner into the hallway.

The end is near.
May you gently glide over the Queen City
Toward the space of ultimate peace.

When My Time Comes

I am here…
Witnessing.

Dying is different for each person.
Why does struggle have to be a part of this?
How much does this gentleman not want to die?

When my time comes,
May I lean into and exist in
The peace of gentle dying.
May I bring to the process
An acceptance that guides me,
Soothes me,
Allows the process of dying
To flow…
Unencumbered by fears
And guided by calm.
Aid me in being present
O Mother Death.

Death!
When my time comes,
Swing wide your open door.
Welcome me!
Embrace my physical ending.

CHAPTER 7
Ancestors

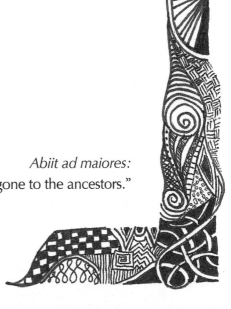

Abiit ad maiores:
"S/he has gone to the ancestors."

Adored Aunt

I look at you in your ninth decade
And I see Suzy
Our children's beloved aunt…
Both of you vibrant and active,
Avid Red Sox fans.
The love you have given over the years,
Reflected in the tender touches
And loving presence
Of your adored nieces and nephews,
Gives me an image
Of how meaningful Suzy's last chapter could be.

Beautifully cared for
After a full life, a long life,
A well-kept woman, I can tell,
Hair well-coiffed even now.

Pass on, adored aunt
Taking all the love
And next-generation gratitude with you.
I can see how cherished you are.
Your time is here.

Mother,
Reach out and be present to this good woman
Just as you did so many new residents
In your treasured shared-living residence.

Bring her to your welcoming dinner table of afterlife
And invite all who loved her
To embrace her in a heavenly welcome.

You Never Know

Oh my... You never know!
A stranger by birth name
In two hours vigil time
Goes from unknown and unfamiliar
To recognized and known.

Upon arrival,
I see an unresponsive cloak of dying.
Yet, when the masks of aging
And never used birth name,
Along with decades of absence
Are erased...
And his pen name is spoken,
I find I am sitting vigil with,
Not just a contemporary of my Dad's,
But a newspaper colleague and friend.

What gifts this anonymous volunteering brings.
I speak to him and reintroduce myself.
A faint response occurs.
I am honored to sit in for Dad
And to pass invisible loving feelings
For him to carry on his journey.

Dad...
Be a spirit that aids his passing.
There is a little something extra in it for you
As he's soul-carrying my loving thoughts to you.

Common Essence

The anniversary of your death, Dad,
And here I sit,
A ten year gap
Between your death
And that of this woman.
You, surrounded by your loving family
After a life of accomplishment
And good fortune;
Her,
Alone in her final hours,
In a body worn out by abusive substances.
Yet, on some level,
We all enter and leave this world
With the simple commonality
Of our core essence,
Entering pure of heart and innocent,
Ready to absorb
All that life holds for us,
And, as we prepare to leave,
Letting go of all that life gave to us,
Each hand played
With the cards that were dealt.

Once More the Unanticipated Gift

A new patient and upon my arrival,
From the foot of the bed
I look and take a deep breath…
It is my grandmother's face I see.
Nanny died forty-three years ago
Forty-three years and ten days.
That beautiful face…
High forehead with lovely facial features.

I never saw my cherished grandmother ill
During those last few hospital months.
I was in Maryland and very pregnant.
My planned pilgrimage home
With our first-born was too late;
We arrived the day after she died.

My grandmother always made me feel special.
When I was ten or eleven
I would walk the three miles into town to visit her,
Sometimes being invited to stay overnight
In her huge downtown Victorian home.
She taught me to play Canasta
And often had a small gift
In her white flower-embossed bureau
To give me as I was leaving.

She was a proud woman and very stylish.
B. Loretto Mulqueen Dower:
A young widow
Who ran her late husband's funeral home
At a time when it was not fashionable
For women to be in business.
Great Uncle Ed was her front man;
In later years her son, Uncle Maurice, her partner.

I adored her
And I feel as if I am with her now.
I stare in disbelief in this moment.
My opportunity to be with my dying grandmother,
To visualize what it might have been like…
The gift of one more chance.

Tears rise…
Forty-three years and here we are together again.
       How fortunate am I?
               How precious is this…

Once more … the unanticipated gift!

We're a Team!

*(I discovered a new relationship with my mother
in the course of sitting this vigil, my family having
done the same for Mother a few short months before.)*

Here's another, Mother…

I sit at this woman's bedside.
Quietly.
I gently touch her hand,
Not wanting to stimulate
The feistiness of her altered mind.

Eighty-eight years of farming
And a dementia'ed death
Is the un-chosen closure
Of a life, hard-worked
Close to the land.
Now, seven breaths,
Then thirty to forty seconds of stillness,
A long life journey ending.

I see you, Mother,
In her one eye that is open, involuntarily,
Just a small slit.
I remember how your eye did that.

I think you're reminding me
That you and I are a team…
Always were.

Here's to your next welcoming assignment!
I'll send; you receive –
And with her comes my love to you…

Ahhh, yes; we're still a team!

Billy Bob

A large muscular burly man
Lies restless, sighing…

To witness your child
Only four decades old…
Oh so young –
Face a relentless cancer
Over a few short months…
What a heart breaker for a mom –
Big bruiser
Being felled by wayward cells.

Remove his fear;
Relieve his pain.
Ancestors – Please embrace him.
Bring him to a place of love and peace.

And, in honoring his arm's tattoo inscription,
We will "Never Forget."

CHAPTER 8

Journey

"Be here now."

RAM DASS

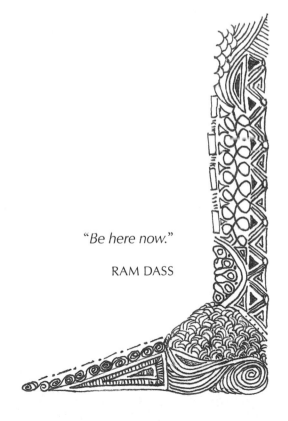

Passionate Living

Tender and jaundiced skin
Encasing weakened and frail contents.
A body mass
Dwindling down to its core.

With today's arrival of a new wheelchair,
This passionate dragonboat racer
Summons the playful energy
To have a wild ride
Inside the house.
"I can do it myself.", you tell me.
You were delightfully out of control!
Soon, your body's empty gas tank
Guides you back to your resting place
On the couch.
Drained.
You select a CD and we listen to music together.

You were a potter;
You shaped clay
From lump to beauty.
Now you are shaping your final days,
One like another,
Differing in pain, fatigue,
Connections and closures,
Putting the final touches on your life.

As with the last firing of a pot
Almost ready to meet its new owner,
You prepare your way
To exit this studio of life
And enter your new life
Fully radiant and whole again;
Passionately, abundantly beautiful.

Magical Mystery

My privilege,
While the world is asleep,
Is to witness final moments –
Labored breath its only action;
A man awaiting transition
From breathless to beyond.

How is it
That these mystery-filled moments
Unite with earliest beginnings,
Blending new born night awakeness
With death's darkened calling?

A door gently opens.
A new life slides through it
Cradled in arms warm and loving,
As across town and ago
Another life slips out
Into the waiting arms of eternity.

Fellow Traveller

Quiet –
Only the sound of oxygen
Bubbling through water.
My choice of soft classical music
Wafts from the player in the background.
I wish I could know your choice.

Handsome man,
Traveling a final journey…
Your past and accomplishments
Are camouflaged
By your unresponsive stillness.
Generic white sheets
And a hospital room
Devoid of personal items
Provide no clues.

For me, your face holds many faces.
I can imagine you
As a respected banker,
A student-loved science teacher
A playful adored grandfather.
What joys did your life hold?
What responsibilities…
What burdens…

I have nothing to go on.
Observation and speculation
Carry no truth.

What I do know, though,
Is that you are my fellow traveler
And you are approaching your destination.
It is a privilege
To travel these last few miles with you.
May your soul have a gentle landing
In a peaceful place of contentment.

Symbolic Imagery

Sweetness in pink,
Whisper soft voice,
Ever the hostess.
"The paper's over there,"
Her welcoming gesture for me.

She is so loved by nieces and nephews,
Her surrogate children.
After 91, a pneumonia
And her frail, bird-like body
Finds it hard to fight,
Yet her spirit has spunk;
She's not ready to let go.

"Are my shoes in the hallway?"
She asks upon waking three different times…
The final time, I ask,
"Are you going somewhere?"
A positive nod and she returns to sleep.

Is this symbolic language, I wonder…
Is she referring to her final voyage?
Her family so hopes she can wait;
Tomorrow her favorite nephew will arrive.

Wait for Joe, her family urges.
Wait for Joe…
He'll be here tomorrow
And you'll have full permission
To let go…
To go…

Your shoes await you in the hallway.

Endings and Beginnings

Cold hands
Mottle on their undersides.

As you rhythmically breathe,
Your seven breaths
Ascend and descend
And then give way to
Thirty seconds of apnea,
A transition
Not unlike labor and birth.
The intervals of labor
Grow shorter with each contraction;
The intervals between breaths
Grow longer in dying.

The end is nearing,
As did one day a beginning.
A color-draining ending
Mirrors color-pinking beginning
As you entered this world,
Each passage
As sacred and momentous as the other.
Anticipation and delight with beginnings;
Blessings and releases with endings…
A long life now has been well lived.

And, as my dear friend Dorrie was fond of saying,
"It's the dash"…
The lifespan that lies between

The inscribed years of birth and death;
The times, the experiences,
The relationships
Hold the substance
By which a life is measured.

Enough

I am an isolated link
Yet, of the basics, I have enough.

Enough information to get me here.
Vt. Respite House .... Name ...Restless... Vigil...

Enough welcome to get me to the right room
"Sure. I'll show you to his room."
"Thank you, Margaret."

Enough reason to be "present"
And enough meaning in these moments
To feel called
To offer respite and relief
To welcome peace
In witnessing one man's final steps
In his journey of life.

But for those who care
Is it enough?
I dare say not.

For when we face the mystery
Of eternal forever,
That which is certain,
That which we grasp,
That which we love
Is never enough.

CHAPTER 9

Close to Heart

SEQUENTIAL POEMS

*By its very nature, vigil sitting is an intimate experience.
The following poems were written about three individuals to
whom I felt very close. I asked for and received permission
from their families to not remove or change their names.*

Soul Peace

Ann #1

Ann, dear Ann…
We share whispers of love and concern
As I sit
Quietly
Breathing with you.

Your life force dwindling,
Closed eyes allow you to stay inward
Seeking your place of peace.

Your daughter's violin in a nearby room
Bows musical maternal love notes,
As you release each breath
With a sound indicating effort.

Find that place of soul peace, Ann.
Enter it deeply – wholly,
Knowing that the love of so many
Embraces your physical presence
And wants you only
In that immersed, safe, rich space of love.

Death's Stillness

*Ann #2: I receive the call that Ann has passed
and her family generously invites me to return.*

The form familiar
Although frail and wasted...
Your angular, chiseled features
Freed from pain and fear.
Still.

The outline of spindly legs
Under loving white knitted coverlet...
You resting in the home you loved
For all of your married years.
Tranquil.

I lay my hand
As I had done hours before
On your emaciated, now cooled arm.
Empty.

The husk of your being,
Being simply the container,
Rests lifeless, yet beautiful...
A lifetime aura of beauty surrounds you.
Magnificent...

Your soul, your essence,
Still feels present throughout this room.
Perhaps the Buddhist belief is true;
It takes time.
Time for the spirit to leave the body.
How can one know?
Peaceful.

The swallows,
Swooping and circling outside the open window,
Have come to welcome your spirit,
To guide and lift you to your new universe of ubiquity.
Eternal.

May your spirit be present
At times both meaningful and unexpected
In the lives and hearts of your dearest, Ann.
Always.

The Fullness of Giving

Ann #3: And later that evening, at home…

I am in recovery,
Body fatigue felt to the bone.
My emotional resources,
Drawn and quartered,
Have been given in such entirety
That I am caught by surprise –

Whoa!
Was I not aware of what I was giving?
Perhaps not; certainly not entirely.
I now see that I was in my truest self.
Being fully in the moment came easily…
Opening myself to whatever was present,
Giving in its purest form…

And what allowed that?
What was in the environment
That brought me to that place
Of safety, of purest emotional honestly?

I dare say…
Expressed appreciation.
Absence of judgment.
Trust.
Belief in me.

Such beautiful gifts,
Deeply appreciated,
Magnified my ability to give.

Proxy

Gary #1

I pretend as I sit
In this silence of darkness,
In the rising shadow of death,
That this gentleman is Gary

No, not pretend –
That's not what I mean.
That feels disrespectful.

It is that I am thinking about Gary
And dedicate these few after-midnight hours
Of privilege, of presence,
To the waning, life-loving spirit
Of cousin Nancy's dear husband.

May some kind Floridian,
Who is able to be a heart presence,
Do the same thing for Gary
Who lays dying in a hospice in Florida.

Be my proxy.
Please stand in.
Bear witness in the name of family,
In the name of love.

Surrogates in a Darkened Room

Gary #2

I enter to the rhythmic whirring
Of an air-moving fan
Offering relief for breathlessness
In these late night hours of darkness.

The love and commitment of many
Is evident throughout this room.
One cherished friend at her bedside,
Bearing witness for a whole community,
Is overcome by fatigue
As she sits with upper body draped over bed pillows
Watching medication-calmed breathing.

With her head slumped sideways on her pillow
We watch her chest rising, then dropping upon exhale,
These last moments of life
The effort of breath-sustaining existence
Being all she can manage.

Memories of better times are shared…
Twenty years of companioning,
Being there for each other.
That remains unchanged.

Our warm hands touch.
A fatigued, gracious smile appears on her face.
The outstretched futon
Beckons her headachy body –
"Rest now, while I am here," I offer…
"*But…*"
"I will awaken you if anything changes."

I sit – present in a silent vigil
Witnessing one more life passing…
A body's machinery slowly winding down.
This honorable task has special meaning tonight
As I am unable, because of distance,
To sit with my cousin Gary, dying in Florida.

May two peaceful souls meet
In the ultimate place of peace,
That which lies on the edge of forever.

Delta Dawn

Jenny #1

"I have the thoughts
But my hands are too tired to write,"
I am told by this young mother.
The request: Be her hands.
Write whatever she is needing done.
Her time is short.

Jaundiced and fighting frequent nausea
Is this gentle, sweet spirit.
"I began journaling in sixth grade," she tells me.
"I won a contest and a journal was the prize!"
"I went back when I was in college
And told the teacher, who was still teaching,
How journaling became such an important part of my
life."

I am in awe…
Integrity, courage and honesty
Are an integral part of this young woman,
Along with a deep faith in her god.

We make plans…
I make a "Private: We're Writing" sign for her door.
I leave a tablet at her bedside for her to write thoughts.
We set my next visit for the following day…
And we begin…

One day, while we were writing,
The Noyana Hospice chorus arrived at her door
Offering to sing for Jenny.
She timidly accepted and,
With me sitting on the bed with her,
We were serenaded with beautiful tones and voices.
"Is there anything else you'd like us to sing?" they asked.
Her soft voice replied,
"Do you know Delta Dawn?"
Two of the six people did and soon all were joining in.

I had never listened closely to the words of that song…
And did I hear you say,
He was a-meeting you here today,
To take you to his mansion in the sky…

I'll never hear that song without thinking of you, Jenny.

Jenny in Paradise

Jenny #2

I enter and see calm.
Gentle, soft music plays
As you lay upright, basin nearby,
Your sallow, yellow skin
Encasing dropped eyelids and lip.
You sleep.

I whisper, "It's Pam. I'll sit with you, Jenny."
You stir, look at me, and softly say "Hi"
I kiss your forehead, tell you to sleep;
That your journey is near completion.

We had just three weeks, it turned out,
With an agreement that tears were okay…
For both of us.
She dictated and I wrote…
Letters to her parents, her children
Her husband and her best friends.
I bought beautiful paper and envelopes
On which to put her precious words.
I chose an attractive font and typed them;
She was barely able to sign them.
I tied them with a silken ribbon
For her to give to her husband.
They were to go into their safety deposit box for now.

This passive and brave work of dying...
"Going to a more beautiful place," you said,
As I witnessed and learned from you:
Acceptance – when no hope for cure
Commitment – to family and loved friends
Generosity – of spirit so full
Openness – the gift to me each visit
Closure – completed with class and with courage.

We opened our souls to each other
With unconditional acceptance;
I'll always be grateful
For the tender time spent together.

You're a jewel, Delta Dawn!
Be free, oh sweet spirit...
Fly over the ocean and the lands.
Sprinkle love on your children.
You're leaving a piece of your indomitable spirit
With each of us who love you.

EPILOGUE

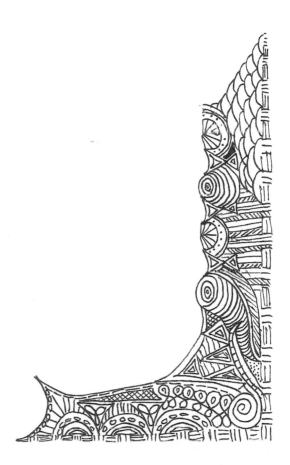

Important Work This Dying

Important work this dying,
Lying in wait
Existing
Sleep-closed eyes
Or unresponsive stares.

What goes on?
Is it dreaming? Or oblivion?
Does a mind chatter?
Or does it float on the waves of immeasurable
endlessness?

When the times comes,
Will I have the courage to say:
Let me do this the best way I can.
Let me go through my dying process
In as conscious and intentional a way as is possible.
I want to suck the marrow out of life…
To lift high the blinds on life's windows
And embrace the warmth of sunlight;
Absorb the beauty of the night sky.

I can do it if you'll be there with me,
As I also face storms and clouds.
Let's be courageous together
As I walk my journey to forevermore.

Author Biography

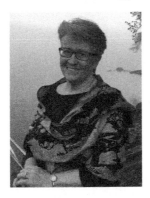

Pamela Heinrich MacPherson has been a community advocate for end-of-life care for over three decades. A native of Burlington, Vermont, her first understanding and respect for dying and death came from her maternal grandmother, one of the area's early female professionals and funeral directors.

In 1964, Pam graduated from the Jeanne Mance School of Nursing, where she was drawn to end-of-life care issues. She later received training as a hospice volunteer and served as Hospice Volunteer Coordinator for the Visiting Nurse Association of Chittenden and Grand Isle Counties (VNA) from 1988-2004, a position to which she brought passion and dedication.

Retirement from the VNA in 2004 allowed her to give more time and energy to community resources related to quality care at the end of life. Sitting vigil with dying individuals in their home, at Vermont Respite House or in the hospital holds life's deepest meaning for her. As a founding member, Pam's involvement with VNA's Madison-Deane Initiative (MDI) has spanned two decades. MDI is an organization that seeks to change the face of dying through education of health care professionals and the general public.

Pam is married to Bruce R. MacPherson, M.D., a retired pathologist and professor at the University of Vermont College of Medicine. They have three grown children and reside in South Burlington, Vermont.

CPSIA information can be obtained
at www.ICGtesting.com
Printed in the USA
BVOW08s0758201116
468399BV00001B/79/P